DR. BARBARA EASY MUCUS CLEANSE

Discover Dr. Barbara's simple mucus cleanse: Transform your health with easy-to-follow steps and recipes for natural wellness and vitality

Charlos Luz

Table of Contents

COPYRIGHT © 2023

CHAPTER ONE

Introduction to Dr. Barbara's Gentle Approach to Mucus Cleansing

In recent years, there has been a growing interest in holistic health practices, including methods aimed at cleansing the body of toxins and impurities. Among these practices, mucus cleansing has gained attention for its potential to improve overall well-being by targeting the removal of excess mucus from the body. Dr. Barbara's gentle approach to mucus cleansing offers a comprehensive and nuanced perspective on this topic, emphasizing the importance of gentle methods that support the body's natural processes without causing undue stress or discomfort.

Understanding Mucus and Its Role in the Body

Before delving into Dr. Barbara's approach to mucus cleansing, it's essential to understand the role that mucus plays in the body. Mucus is a viscous fluid produced by mucous membranes throughout the body, including the respiratory, digestive, and reproductive systems. It serves several vital functions, including lubricating and protecting tissues, trapping foreign particles and pathogens, and facilitating the movement of materials within the body.

In a healthy state, mucus production is balanced, providing necessary protection without causing congestion or discomfort. However, factors such as poor diet, environmental toxins, stress, and certain medical conditions can disrupt this balance, leading to excessive mucus production or thickened mucus that becomes difficult to clear from the body.

The Importance of Gentle Cleansing Methods

Dr. Barbara's approach to mucus cleansing emphasizes the use of gentle methods that support the body's natural detoxification processes without causing harm or discomfort. Unlike more aggressive cleansing protocols that may involve harsh chemicals, extreme dietary restrictions, or invasive procedures, Dr. Barbara's methods prioritize the maintenance of overall health and well-being.

Gentle cleansing techniques focus on supporting the body's natural detoxification organs, such as the liver, kidneys, and lymphatic system, which play crucial roles in filtering and eliminating toxins from the body. By promoting optimal function of these organs through dietary and lifestyle interventions, gentle cleansing can help restore balance and alleviate symptoms associated with excess mucus production.

Key Principles of Dr. Barbara's Approach

Dr. Barbara's gentle approach to mucus cleansing is rooted in several key principles that guide her recommendations for supporting optimal health and well-being:

1. **Nutrient-Rich Diet:** Central to Dr. Barbara's approach is the emphasis on a nutrient-rich diet that provides essential vitamins, minerals, antioxidants, and phytonutrients necessary for cellular function and detoxification. A diet rich in whole, plant-based foods, including fruits, vegetables, whole grains, legumes, nuts, and seeds, can help nourish the body and support its natural detoxification processes.

2. **Hydration:** Adequate hydration is essential for maintaining healthy mucous membranes and supporting the body's detoxification pathways. Dr. Barbara recommends drinking plenty of water throughout the day to help flush toxins from the body and keep mucous membranes hydrated and functioning optimally.

3. **Supporting Detoxification Organs:** Dr. Barbara's approach includes strategies for supporting the liver, kidneys, and lymphatic system, which are primary organs involved in detoxification. This may involve incorporating specific foods and herbs known for their detoxifying properties, such as dandelion root, milk thistle, turmeric, and cilantro, into the diet.

4. **Stress Management:** Chronic stress can impair the body's detoxification processes and contribute to mucus imbalance. Dr. Barbara emphasizes the importance of stress management techniques, such as mindfulness, meditation, yoga, and deep breathing exercises, for promoting relaxation and supporting overall health.

5. **Gentle Detoxification Practices:** Rather than harsh cleanses or extreme fasting protocols, Dr. Barbara advocates for gentle detoxification practices that support the body's natural rhythms and processes. This may include periodic fasting, juice cleansing, herbal teas, and other methods that promote detoxification without causing undue stress or discomfort.

Benefits of Dr. Barbara's Gentle Approach

The benefits of Dr. Barbara's gentle approach to mucus cleansing are manifold and encompass not only improved respiratory health but also enhanced overall well-being. By prioritizing gentle methods that support the body's natural detoxification processes, individuals may experience the following benefits:

1. **Improved Respiratory Function:** Excess mucus in the respiratory tract can lead to symptoms such as congestion, coughing, and difficulty breathing. By promoting the removal of excess mucus through gentle cleansing techniques,

individuals may experience improved respiratory function and reduced respiratory symptoms.

2. **Enhanced Digestive Health:** Mucus imbalance in the digestive tract can contribute to symptoms such as bloating, gas, constipation, and diarrhea. Gentle cleansing methods can help support digestive health by promoting optimal function of the gastrointestinal tract and supporting the elimination of toxins and waste products.

3. **Increased Energy and Vitality:** By removing toxins and supporting the body's natural detoxification processes, gentle cleansing practices can help increase energy levels and vitality. Many individuals report feeling lighter, more energized, and mentally clear after completing a gentle cleansing protocol.

4. **Immune Support:** The immune system relies on a healthy balance of mucus production to defend against pathogens and foreign invaders. By promoting optimal immune function through gentle cleansing methods, individuals may experience enhanced immune support and reduced susceptibility to illness.

5. **Overall Well-Being:** Perhaps most importantly, Dr. Barbara's gentle approach to mucus cleansing supports overall well-being by promoting balance and harmony within the body. By prioritizing gentle methods that respect the body's

natural rhythms and processes, individuals can achieve lasting improvements in their health and vitality.

Conclusion

In conclusion, Dr. Barbara's gentle approach to mucus cleansing offers a comprehensive and nuanced perspective on this important aspect of holistic health. By prioritizing gentle methods that support the body's natural detoxification processes, Dr. Barbara helps individuals achieve optimal health and well-being without resorting to harsh cleanses or extreme protocols. With a focus on nutrient-rich foods, hydration, stress management, and gentle detoxification practices, Dr. Barbara's approach empowers individuals to take control of their health and cultivate balance and harmony within the body.

CHAPTER TWO

Understanding Mucus and Its Impact on Health: Dr. Barbara's Insights

Mucus is often misunderstood and overlooked in discussions about health and wellness, yet its impact on the body is profound. Dr. Barbara brings a wealth of insights into the role of mucus in health and disease, highlighting its importance in maintaining optimal physiological function and the potential consequences of mucus imbalance. In this exploration, we delve into Dr. Barbara's perspectives on mucus and its intricate relationship with health.

The Role of Mucus in the Body

Mucus is a complex mixture of water, proteins, antibodies, and glycoproteins produced by mucous membranes throughout the body. It serves multiple critical functions, including:

1. **Protection:** Mucus acts as a physical barrier, trapping pathogens, allergens, and other foreign particles before they can enter the body. This protective function is particularly crucial in the respiratory and digestive systems, where mucous membranes line the airways and gastrointestinal tract.

2. **Lubrication:** Mucus lubricates and moisturizes tissues, preventing dryness and irritation. In the respiratory system,

for example, mucus helps keep the airways moist, facilitating efficient breathing and protecting against irritation from airborne pollutants.

3. **Transport:** Mucus aids in the movement of materials within the body, such as food through the digestive tract and sperm through the female reproductive tract. In the respiratory system, cilia—hair-like structures embedded in the mucous membrane—beat rhythmically to propel mucus and trapped particles out of the airways.

Impact of Mucus Imbalance on Health

While mucus plays essential roles in maintaining health, imbalances in mucus production or composition can have significant implications for health and well-being. Dr. Barbara highlights several ways in which mucus imbalance can impact health:

1. **Respiratory Disorders:** Excessive mucus production or thickened mucus can contribute to respiratory conditions such as asthma, chronic bronchitis, and sinusitis. In these conditions, mucus may become thick and viscous, making it difficult to clear from the airways and leading to symptoms such as coughing, wheezing, and difficulty breathing.

2. **Digestive Issues:** Mucus imbalance in the digestive tract can contribute to gastrointestinal problems such as acid reflux, irritable bowel syndrome (IBS), and inflammatory bowel

disease (IBD). Excessive mucus production may interfere with digestion and nutrient absorption, leading to symptoms such as bloating, abdominal pain, and diarrhea.

3. **Immune Dysfunction:** Disruptions in mucus production or composition can compromise the immune system's ability to defend against pathogens and foreign invaders. Mucus serves as a barrier against infection, trapping bacteria, viruses, and other pathogens before they can enter the body. Imbalances in mucus production may weaken this protective barrier, increasing susceptibility to infections and illness.

4. **Allergic Reactions:** Mucus imbalance can contribute to allergic reactions and respiratory allergies such as hay fever and allergic asthma. In allergic individuals, exposure to allergens triggers an immune response that leads to inflammation and increased mucus production in the respiratory tract, resulting in symptoms such as sneezing, nasal congestion, and itching.

Dr. Barbara's Insights on Mucus Cleansing

Given the critical role of mucus in health and disease, Dr. Barbara emphasizes the importance of maintaining mucus balance through gentle cleansing practices. Rather than targeting mucus directly, Dr. Barbara's approach focuses on supporting the body's natural detoxification processes and promoting overall health and well-being. Key insights from Dr. Barbara include:

1. **Nutrient-Rich Diet:** A diet rich in fruits, vegetables, whole grains, and lean proteins provides essential nutrients necessary for optimal mucus production and function. Dr. Barbara recommends avoiding processed foods, refined sugars, and excessive dairy, which can contribute to mucus imbalance and inflammation.

2. **Hydration:** Adequate hydration is crucial for maintaining healthy mucous membranes and supporting mucus production. Dr. Barbara advises drinking plenty of water throughout the day to keep mucous membranes moist and facilitate the movement of mucus within the body.

3. **Stress Management:** Chronic stress can disrupt mucus balance and weaken the immune system, making individuals more susceptible to infections and illness. Dr. Barbara recommends stress management techniques such as mindfulness, meditation, and deep breathing exercises to promote relaxation and support overall health.

4. **Gentle Detoxification Practices:** Rather than aggressive cleansing protocols, Dr. Barbara advocates for gentle detoxification practices that support the body's natural detoxification pathways. This may include incorporating

detoxifying foods and herbs into the diet, such as leafy greens, cruciferous vegetables, and dandelion root.

5. **Individualized Approach:** Dr. Barbara emphasizes the importance of personalized care and tailoring cleansing protocols to individual needs and preferences. What works for one person may not be suitable for another, and it's essential to listen to your body and adjust your approach accordingly.

Conclusion

In conclusion, Dr. Barbara's insights into mucus and its impact on health underscore the importance of maintaining mucus balance for overall well-being. By understanding the role of mucus in the body and its potential implications for health, individuals can take proactive steps to support mucus health through gentle cleansing practices and lifestyle interventions. Through a holistic approach that prioritizes nutrition, hydration, stress management, and gentle detoxification, individuals can optimize mucus function and promote optimal health and vitality.

CHAPTER THREE

The Basics of Herbal Mucus Cleansing: Simple Steps to Clearing Congestion

Herbal mucus cleansing offers a natural and holistic approach to clearing congestion and promoting respiratory health. By harnessing the therapeutic properties of various herbs, individuals can support the body's natural detoxification processes and alleviate symptoms associated with excess mucus production. In this guide, we explore the basics of herbal mucus cleansing and provide simple steps for clearing congestion effectively.

Understanding Herbal Mucus Cleansing

Herbal mucus cleansing involves the use of medicinal herbs to support respiratory health and promote the removal of excess mucus from the body. These herbs contain compounds that possess expectorant, decongestant, and anti-inflammatory properties, making them valuable allies in addressing respiratory congestion and related symptoms.

When used correctly, herbal mucus cleansing can help:

1. **Loosen and expel mucus:** Expectorant herbs help thin mucus, making it easier to expel from the respiratory tract.

2. **Reduce inflammation:** Anti-inflammatory herbs help soothe inflamed mucous membranes, relieving irritation and discomfort.

3. **Support immune function:** Many herbs have immune-boosting properties that help strengthen the body's defenses against respiratory infections.

Key Herbs for Mucus Cleansing

Several herbs are commonly used in herbal mucus cleansing preparations due to their beneficial effects on respiratory health. Some of the key herbs include:

1. **Eucalyptus:** Eucalyptus is renowned for its decongestant properties and its ability to open up the airways. Inhalation of eucalyptus oil vapors can help clear nasal congestion and relieve respiratory symptoms.

2. **Peppermint:** Peppermint contains menthol, which acts as a natural decongestant and bronchodilator. Peppermint tea or steam inhalation with peppermint oil can help soothe respiratory congestion and promote easier breathing.

3. **Ginger:** Ginger is prized for its anti-inflammatory and expectorant properties. Consuming ginger tea or adding fresh ginger to meals can help reduce inflammation in the respiratory tract and promote the expulsion of mucus.

4. **Licorice:** Licorice root has demulcent properties, meaning it forms a soothing film over mucous membranes, helping to relieve irritation and inflammation. Licorice tea or lozenges can help soothe sore throats and calm coughs.

5. **Thyme:** Thyme contains thymol, a compound with powerful antimicrobial properties. Thyme tea or steam inhalation with thyme oil can help fight respiratory infections and loosen stubborn mucus.

Simple Steps to Herbal Mucus Cleansing

Here are some simple steps to incorporate herbal mucus cleansing into your routine:

1. **Stay Hydrated:** Drink plenty of water throughout the day to keep mucous membranes hydrated and support the body's natural detoxification processes.

2. **Steam Inhalation:** Add a few drops of essential oils such as eucalyptus, peppermint, or thyme to a bowl of hot water. Cover your head with a towel and inhale the steam for 5-10 minutes to help clear nasal congestion and loosen mucus.

3. **Herbal Teas:** Drink herbal teas made from mucus-cleansing herbs such as ginger, licorice, peppermint, or thyme. Steep the herbs in hot water for 5-10 minutes, then strain and enjoy. You can also add honey or lemon for additional soothing benefits.

4. **Herbal Supplements:** Consider taking herbal supplements formulated specifically for respiratory health and mucus cleansing. Look for products containing a combination of mucus-clearing herbs for comprehensive support.

5. **Nasal Irrigation:** Use a saline nasal spray or neti pot to rinse your nasal passages and flush out excess mucus and allergens. This can help relieve nasal congestion and improve breathing.

Precautions and Considerations

While herbal mucus cleansing can be beneficial for many individuals, it's essential to exercise caution and consult with a healthcare professional, especially if you have any underlying health conditions or are taking medications. Some herbs may interact with certain medications or exacerbate existing health issues, so it's crucial to seek personalized advice before starting any herbal regimen.

Additionally, if you experience severe or persistent respiratory symptoms, such as difficulty breathing, chest pain, or high fever, seek medical attention promptly, as these could be signs of a more serious underlying condition.

Conclusion

Herbal mucus cleansing offers a natural and effective approach to clearing congestion and supporting respiratory health. By incorporating mucus-clearing herbs into your daily routine through teas, steam inhalation, and supplements, you can help loosen and expel excess mucus from the body, alleviate respiratory symptoms, and promote overall well-being. Remember to stay hydrated, consult with a healthcare professional as needed, and listen to your body's signals to ensure safe and effective mucus cleansing.

CHAPTER FOUR

Preparing for Your Cleanse: Getting Ready Mentally and Physically

Embarking on a cleanse, whether it's a mucus cleanse or any other type, requires preparation both mentally and physically. Taking the time to prepare adequately can help set you up for success and maximize the benefits of your cleanse. In this guide, we'll explore the essential steps to get ready for your cleanse, focusing on both mental and physical readiness.

Mental Preparation

1. **Set Clear Intentions:** Before starting your cleanse, take some time to reflect on why you're doing it and what you hope to achieve. Setting clear intentions can help keep you focused and motivated throughout the process.

2. **Educate Yourself:** Learn about the cleanse you'll be undertaking, including its purpose, potential benefits, and any guidelines or restrictions involved. Understanding the rationale behind the cleanse can help you stay committed and informed as you progress.

3. **Visualize Success:** Spend some time visualizing yourself successfully completing the cleanse and reaping the benefits of improved health and vitality. Visualizing success can help

build confidence and reinforce your commitment to the process.

4. **Address Any Concerns:** If you have any concerns or reservations about the cleanse, don't hesitate to address them. Talk to a healthcare professional or seek guidance from a trusted source to address any questions or uncertainties you may have.

5. **Practice Mindfulness:** Cultivate a mindset of mindfulness and self-awareness as you prepare for your cleanse. Pay attention to your thoughts, emotions, and physical sensations, and approach the cleanse with curiosity and openness.

Physical Preparation

1. **Gradually Reduce Stimulants:** If you consume caffeine, alcohol, or other stimulants regularly, consider gradually reducing your intake in the days leading up to your cleanse. This can help minimize withdrawal symptoms and make the transition smoother.

2. **Hydrate:** Start hydrating well in advance of your cleanse by drinking plenty of water throughout the day. Proper hydration is essential for supporting detoxification and maintaining overall health.

3. **Cleanse Your Environment:** Take some time to clean and declutter your living space, including your kitchen and pantry. Removing temptations and creating a clean, organized environment can help support your cleanse and minimize distractions.

4. **Meal Planning:** Plan your meals ahead of time to ensure you have plenty of nourishing foods on hand during your cleanse. Stock up on fresh fruits, vegetables, whole grains, and other cleanse-friendly foods to make meal preparation easier.

5. **Gather Supplies:** Depending on the type of cleanse you'll be undertaking, gather any supplies or equipment you'll need in advance. This may include herbal teas, supplements, juicing ingredients, or detoxifying herbs.

General Tips

1. **Set Realistic Expectations:** Understand that cleansing is a process, and results may not be immediate or dramatic. Set realistic expectations for yourself and focus on progress rather than perfection.

2. **Listen to Your Body:** Pay attention to how your body responds to the cleanse and adjust your approach accordingly. If you experience discomfort or adverse reactions, don't hesitate to modify or discontinue the cleanse as needed.

3. **Seek Support:** Enlist the support of friends, family members, or online communities who can provide encouragement and accountability during your cleanse. Having a support system can make the journey more enjoyable and rewarding.

4. **Practice Self-Care:** Prioritize self-care activities such as meditation, gentle exercise, and relaxation techniques during your cleanse. Taking care of your physical and emotional well-being is essential for a successful cleanse.

5. **Celebrate Your Progress:** Celebrate your achievements and milestones along the way, no matter how small. Acknowledge the effort you're putting into your cleanse and celebrate the positive changes you're experiencing.

By preparing mentally and physically for your cleanse, you can set yourself up for a successful and fulfilling experience. Remember to approach the process with patience, openness, and self-compassion, and trust in your body's ability to heal and rejuvenate through the cleansing process.

CHAPTER FIVE

Day 1: Starting Your Cleanse with Easy-to-Prepare Herbal Remedies

Congratulations on taking the first step towards a healthier you by starting your cleanse journey! Day 1 marks the beginning of your cleanse, and it's essential to ease into the process gradually while nourishing your body with gentle, herbal remedies. In this guide, we'll explore some easy-to-prepare herbal remedies that will support your cleanse and help you feel refreshed and rejuvenated from the start.

Morning: Herbal Detox Tea

Start your day with a soothing cup of herbal detox tea to kickstart your cleanse and support your body's natural detoxification processes. Here's a simple recipe to try:

Ingredients:

- 1 teaspoon dried dandelion root

- 1 teaspoon dried burdock root

- 1 teaspoon dried nettle leaf

- 1 teaspoon dried ginger root

- 1 teaspoon dried peppermint leaf

- 4 cups water

Instructions:

1. In a small saucepan, bring the water to a boil.

2. Add the dried herbs to the boiling water and reduce the heat to low.

3. Simmer the herbs for 10-15 minutes, allowing the flavors to infuse into the water.

4. Remove the saucepan from the heat and let the tea cool slightly.

5. Strain the tea into a mug and enjoy it warm.

This herbal detox tea is packed with cleansing herbs like dandelion, burdock, nettle, ginger, and peppermint, which help support liver function, promote digestion, and eliminate toxins from the body.

Midday: Green Smoothie Cleanse

For a refreshing and nutrient-packed midday cleanse, try a green smoothie made with cleansing ingredients like leafy greens, fruits, and herbs. Here's a simple recipe to try:

Ingredients:

- 2 cups spinach or kale

- 1 ripe banana

- 1/2 cup fresh or frozen berries (such as blueberries or strawberries)

- 1 tablespoon fresh lemon juice

- 1 tablespoon fresh ginger, peeled and grated

- 1 cup coconut water or almond milk

- Handful of ice cubes

Instructions:

1. Place all the ingredients in a blender.

2. Blend until smooth and creamy, adding more liquid if needed to reach your desired consistency.

3. Pour the smoothie into a glass and enjoy immediately.

This green smoothie is rich in antioxidants, vitamins, and minerals, which help support detoxification, boost energy levels, and promote overall well-being.

Evening: Herbal Steam Inhalation

End your day with a relaxing herbal steam inhalation to clear your respiratory passages and promote deep relaxation. Here's how to do it:

Ingredients:

- 2 cups hot water

- 2-3 drops eucalyptus essential oil

- 2-3 drops peppermint essential oil

- Towel

Instructions:

1. Boil the water in a large pot.

2. Remove the pot from the heat and add the eucalyptus and peppermint essential oils.

3. Place the pot on a stable surface and sit comfortably with your face positioned above the steam.

4. Drape a towel over your head to create a tent, trapping the steam inside.

5. Close your eyes and breathe deeply, inhaling the aromatic steam for 5-10 minutes.

6. Afterward, pat your face dry with a clean towel and follow up with your evening skincare routine.

This herbal steam inhalation helps open up your airways, relieve congestion, and promote relaxation, making it the perfect way to unwind and prepare for a restful night's sleep.

Conclusion

Day 1 of your cleanse sets the tone for the rest of your journey, and incorporating these easy-to-prepare herbal remedies can help you start on the right foot. Remember to listen to your body, stay hydrated, and nourish yourself with nutrient-dense foods and beverages throughout the day. With each sip and inhale, you're supporting your body's natural detoxification processes and paving the way for a healthier, revitalized you. Cheers to a successful cleanse journey!

CHAPTER SIX

Days 2-3: Continuing the Cleanse with Gentle Herbs and Nutrient-Rich Foods

As you progress through your cleanse journey, days 2-3 are crucial for maintaining momentum and nourishing your body with gentle herbs and nutrient-rich foods. These days are an opportunity to deepen your cleanse experience while supporting your body's natural detoxification processes. In this guide, we'll explore how to continue your cleanse with a focus on gentle herbs and nourishing foods to promote overall well-being.

Day 2: Herbal Infusions for Detoxification

On day 2 of your cleanse, incorporate herbal infusions into your routine to support detoxification and replenish your body with essential nutrients. Herbal infusions are a simple and effective way to harness the therapeutic properties of cleansing herbs. Here's how to prepare them:

Morning: Nettle Tea

Nettle tea is a powerhouse of nutrients and has diuretic properties that support kidney function and promote detoxification. To prepare nettle tea:

Ingredients:

- 1 tablespoon dried nettle leaves

- 1 cup hot water

Instructions:

1. Place the dried nettle leaves in a teapot or mug.

2. Pour hot water over the nettle leaves.

3. Steep for 5-10 minutes, then strain.

4. Drink nettle tea in the morning to kickstart your day and support detoxification.

Midday: Dandelion Root Tea

Dandelion root tea is renowned for its liver-cleansing properties and helps stimulate bile production, aiding in the elimination of toxins from the body. To prepare dandelion root tea:

Ingredients:

- 1 tablespoon dried dandelion root
- 1 cup hot water

Instructions:

1. Place the dried dandelion root in a teapot or mug.

2. Pour hot water over the dandelion root.

3. Steep for 10-15 minutes, then strain.

4. Enjoy dandelion root tea midday to support liver detoxification and digestion.

Evening: Chamomile Tea

Chamomile tea is known for its calming and soothing properties, making it the perfect choice for winding down in the evening. Additionally, chamomile supports digestion and promotes relaxation, essential for a restful night's sleep. To prepare chamomile tea:

Ingredients:

- 1 tablespoon dried chamomile flowers

- 1 cup hot water

Instructions:

1. Place the dried chamomile flowers in a teapot or mug.

2. Pour hot water over the chamomile flowers.

3. Steep for 5-10 minutes, then strain.

4. Enjoy chamomile tea in the evening to relax and unwind.

Day 3: Nourishing Meals for Sustained Energy

On day 3 of your cleanse, focus on nourishing your body with nutrient-rich meals to sustain energy levels and support overall well-being. Incorporate a variety of whole foods, including fruits, vegetables, whole grains, legumes, and healthy fats, to provide essential vitamins, minerals, and antioxidants. Here are some meal ideas to inspire you:

Breakfast: Green Smoothie Bowl

Blend together spinach, kale, avocado, banana, and almond milk to create a creamy green smoothie bowl. Top with fresh berries, sliced almonds, and a sprinkle of chia seeds for added texture and nutrients.

Lunch: Quinoa Salad

Combine cooked quinoa with diced cucumber, cherry tomatoes, bell peppers, avocado, and chickpeas. Drizzle with a lemon-tahini dressing and garnish with fresh herbs like parsley or cilantro.

Snack: Sliced Apple with Almond Butter

Slice an apple and spread each slice with almond butter for a satisfying and nutrient-rich snack. The combination of fiber, vitamins, and healthy fats will keep you feeling full and energized until your next meal.

Dinner: Roasted Vegetable Buddha Bowl

Roast a variety of colorful vegetables such as sweet potatoes, Brussels sprouts, carrots, and cauliflower until tender and caramelized. Serve over a bed of cooked quinoa or brown rice and drizzle with tahini sauce for a nourishing and satisfying meal.

Conclusion

Days 2-3 of your cleanse are an opportunity to deepen your detoxification experience while nourishing your body with gentle herbs and nutrient-rich foods. By incorporating herbal infusions into your routine and focusing on nourishing meals, you can support your body's natural detoxification processes and promote overall well-being. Remember to listen to your body's cues, stay hydrated, and practice self-care throughout your cleanse journey. With each sip and bite, you're supporting your body's journey toward optimal health and vitality.

CHAPTER SEVEN

Day 4: Enhancing Detoxification and Supporting Your Body's Natural Processes

As you progress into day 4 of your cleanse, it's time to focus on enhancing detoxification and supporting your body's natural processes. This day is an opportunity to deepen your cleanse experience and promote overall well-being through targeted detoxification practices and nourishing self-care. In this guide, we'll explore strategies to enhance detoxification and support your body's natural processes on day 4 of your cleanse.

Morning: Lemon Water Detox

Start your day with a simple yet powerful detox ritual by drinking a glass of warm lemon water. Lemon water helps alkalize the body, stimulate digestion, and support liver function, making it an excellent choice for enhancing detoxification. Here's how to prepare it:

Ingredients:

- 1 cup warm water

- Juice of half a lemon

Instructions:

1. Heat water until warm but not boiling.

2. Squeeze the juice of half a lemon into a cup of warm water.

3. Stir well and drink first thing in the morning on an empty stomach.

Midday: Herbal Lymphatic Support

Support your body's lymphatic system, which plays a crucial role in detoxification, with herbal lymphatic support. Certain herbs, such as cleavers and calendula, help stimulate lymphatic flow and support the body's natural detoxification processes. Consider preparing an herbal infusion or enjoying a lymphatic-supporting herbal tea midday to promote lymphatic drainage and detoxification.

Evening: Detoxifying Bath

End your day with a relaxing and detoxifying bath to promote deep relaxation and support detoxification. Epsom salt baths are particularly beneficial for detoxification, as Epsom salts contain magnesium sulfate, which helps draw toxins out of the body and promote relaxation. Here's how to prepare a detoxifying bath:

Ingredients:

- 1-2 cups Epsom salts

- 10-15 drops of essential oils (such as lavender, eucalyptus, or peppermint)

Instructions:

1. Fill your bathtub with warm water.

2. Add 1-2 cups of Epsom salts to the bathwater and stir until dissolved.

3. Add 10-15 drops of your chosen essential oils to the bathwater and swirl to disperse.

4. Soak in the bath for 20-30 minutes, allowing the salts and essential oils to promote detoxification and relaxation.

Throughout the Day: Hydration and Nutrient-Rich Foods

Stay hydrated throughout the day by drinking plenty of water and herbal teas to support detoxification and promote overall well-being. Focus on consuming nutrient-rich foods such as fruits, vegetables, whole grains, and lean proteins to provide essential vitamins, minerals, and antioxidants to support your body's natural detoxification processes. Incorporate detoxifying foods like leafy greens, cruciferous vegetables, berries, and fresh herbs into your meals to maximize detoxification and promote optimal health.

Conclusion

Day 4 of your cleanse is an opportunity to deepen your detoxification experience and support your body's natural processes. By incorporating simple yet effective detox rituals such as lemon water, herbal lymphatic support, and a detoxifying bath into your day, you can enhance detoxification and promote overall well-being. Remember to stay hydrated, nourish yourself with nutrient-rich foods, and listen to your body's cues throughout the day. With each detoxifying practice, you're supporting your body's journey toward optimal health and vitality.

CHAPTER EIGHT

Day 5: Rejuvenation and Renewal as Your Cleanse Progresses

As you reach day 5 of your cleanse journey, you may start to feel a sense of rejuvenation and renewal as your body continues to detoxify and recalibrate. This day is an opportunity to focus on nurturing yourself and embracing the transformative power of cleansing. In this guide, we'll explore strategies for promoting rejuvenation and renewal on day 5 of your cleanse.

Morning: Gentle Yoga and Meditation

Start your day with a gentle yoga practice and meditation to center yourself and set a positive tone for the day ahead. Gentle yoga poses can help release tension, improve circulation, and support detoxification by stimulating lymphatic flow. Incorporate calming meditation techniques such as deep breathing and mindfulness to promote relaxation and mental clarity.

Midday: Green Juice Cleanse

Nourish your body with a revitalizing green juice cleanse midday to flood your system with essential nutrients and support detoxification. Green juices are rich in chlorophyll, vitamins, minerals, and antioxidants, which help alkalize the body, promote cellular regeneration, and support overall well-being. Consider including ingredients such as kale, spinach, cucumber, celery, lemon, and ginger in your green juice for a refreshing and rejuvenating boost.

Afternoon: Nature Walk or Outdoor Activity

Take advantage of the rejuvenating power of nature by spending time outdoors and connecting with the natural world. Go for a nature walk, hike, or bike ride in a nearby park or nature reserve to recharge your spirit and invigorate your body. Nature has a calming and grounding effect on the mind and body, helping reduce stress and promote overall well-being.

Evening: Self-Care Rituals

Indulge in self-care rituals in the evening to pamper yourself and promote relaxation and renewal. Consider taking a warm bath with Epsom salts and essential oils, practicing gentle self-massage with nourishing body oils, or engaging in a restorative skincare routine with natural, botanical-based products. Set aside time to unwind, reflect, and express gratitude for the progress you've made on your cleanse journey.

Throughout the Day: Hydration and Nourishing Foods

Stay hydrated throughout the day by drinking plenty of water, herbal teas, and hydrating fluids to support detoxification and promote overall well-being. Focus on consuming nourishing foods that provide essential vitamins, minerals, and antioxidants to fuel your body and support your cleanse journey. Incorporate a variety of colorful fruits, vegetables, whole grains, and healthy fats into your meals to maximize nutrition and rejuvenation.

Conclusion

Day 5 of your cleanse is a time for rejuvenation and renewal as you continue to support your body's detoxification process and nourish yourself from the inside out. By incorporating gentle yoga, green juice cleanses, outdoor activities, and self-care rituals into your day, you can promote physical, mental, and emotional well-being. Embrace the transformative power of cleansing and savor the journey as you cultivate a renewed sense of vitality and rejuvenation. With each mindful practice and nourishing choice, you're nurturing your body, mind, and spirit and paving the way for lasting health and wellness.

CHAPTER NINE

Day 6: Finalizing Your Cleanse and Preparing for Reintroducing Foods

As you approach the final day of your cleanse, it's essential to take stock of your progress, celebrate your achievements, and prepare for the transition back to regular eating. Day 6 marks the culmination of your cleanse journey and sets the stage for reintroducing foods in a mindful and nourishing way. In this guide, we'll explore strategies for finalizing your cleanse and preparing for the next phase of your wellness journey.

Morning: Reflection and Gratitude

Start your day with reflection and gratitude for the journey you've embarked on and the progress you've made along the way. Take a few moments to journal about your cleanse experience, noting any insights, challenges, and breakthroughs you've encountered. Cultivate a sense of gratitude for your body's resilience and the opportunity to prioritize your health and well-being.

Midday: Light and Nourishing Meals

As you approach the end of your cleanse, continue to nourish your body with light and nutrient-rich meals that support detoxification and promote overall well-being. Focus on incorporating whole foods such as fruits, vegetables, whole grains, legumes, and lean proteins into your meals to provide essential vitamins, minerals, and antioxidants. Aim for balanced meals that satisfy your hunger while supporting your body's natural detoxification processes.

Afternoon: Gentle Movement and Stretching

Engage in gentle movement and stretching exercises in the afternoon to promote circulation, release tension, and support overall well-being. Consider practicing gentle yoga, tai chi, or qigong to stretch and strengthen your body while promoting relaxation and mental clarity. Focus on connecting with your breath and moving mindfully to honor your body's needs and capabilities.

Evening: Meal Planning and Preparation

Take some time in the evening to plan and prepare for the next phase of your wellness journey, which involves reintroducing foods in a mindful and intentional way. Begin by reviewing your cleanse experience and identifying any foods or food groups you eliminated during the cleanse. Create a meal plan for the upcoming days that includes a variety of nourishing foods and incorporates the foods you plan to reintroduce.

Throughout the Day: Hydration and Self-Care

Stay hydrated throughout the day by drinking plenty of water and herbal teas to support detoxification and promote overall well-being. Prioritize self-care practices such as meditation, deep breathing, and relaxation techniques to reduce stress and promote mental and emotional balance. Listen to your body's cues and honor your need for rest, nourishment, and rejuvenation as you finalize your cleanse journey.

Conclusion

Day 6 of your cleanse is a time for reflection, nourishment, and preparation as you approach the end of your journey and transition back to regular eating. By reflecting on your cleanse experience, nourishing your body with light and nutrient-rich meals, engaging in gentle movement and stretching, and planning for the next phase of your wellness journey, you can set yourself up for success and continue to prioritize your health and well-being. Embrace the lessons learned during your cleanse and carry them forward as you embark on the next chapter of your wellness journey with renewed energy, vitality, and intention.

CHAPTER TEN

Day 7: Completing Your Cleanse and Transitioning Back to Regular Eating

Congratulations on reaching the final day of your cleanse journey! Day 7 marks the completion of your cleanse and the beginning of your transition back to regular eating. As you conclude your cleanse, it's essential to do so mindfully and with intention, ensuring a smooth transition that supports your body's needs and promotes long-term health and well-being. In this guide, we'll explore strategies for completing your cleanse and transitioning back to regular eating in a balanced and nourishing way.

Morning: Gentle Movement and Gratitude Practice

Start your day with gentle movement and a gratitude practice to center yourself and set a positive tone for the day ahead. Engage in gentle yoga, stretching, or a short walk outdoors to promote circulation, release tension, and invigorate your body. Take a few moments to express gratitude for the journey you've embarked on, the lessons learned, and the opportunity to prioritize your health and well-being.

Midday: Reintroducing Whole Foods

As you transition back to regular eating, focus on reintroducing whole foods gradually and mindfully. Begin by incorporating easily digestible foods such as fruits, vegetables, whole grains, legumes, and lean proteins into your meals. Aim for balanced meals that provide essential nutrients while supporting your body's natural detoxification processes. Pay attention to how your body responds to different foods and adjust your diet accordingly.

Afternoon: Hydration and Self-Care

Stay hydrated throughout the day by drinking plenty of water and herbal teas to support detoxification and promote overall well-being. Prioritize self-care practices such as meditation, deep breathing, and relaxation techniques to reduce stress and promote mental and emotional balance. Listen to your body's cues and honor your need for rest, nourishment, and rejuvenation as you transition out of your cleanse.

Evening: Reflecting on Your Cleanse Experience

Take some time in the evening to reflect on your cleanse experience and acknowledge the progress you've made on your wellness journey. Journal about your thoughts, feelings, and insights gained during the cleanse, noting any changes in your energy levels, digestion, mood, or overall well-being. Celebrate your achievements and reaffirm your commitment to prioritizing your health and well-being moving forward.

Throughout the Day: Mindful Eating and Portion Control

As you reintroduce foods back into your diet, practice mindful eating and portion control to maintain balance and prevent overeating. Pay attention to hunger and fullness cues, eat slowly, and savor each bite to enhance satisfaction and digestion. Focus on nourishing your body with nutrient-dense foods while being mindful of portion sizes and maintaining balance in your diet.

NOTE: Day 7 of your cleanse marks the completion of your journey and the beginning of your transition back to regular eating. By completing your cleanse mindfully and with intention, you can set yourself up for long-term success and continue to prioritize your health and well-being. Embrace the lessons learned during your cleanse and carry them forward as you navigate your wellness journey with renewed energy, vitality, and intention. With each mindful choice and nourishing meal, you're empowering yourself to live a life of health, balance, and abundance.

BONUS: SOME ESSENTIAL HERBAL AND NATURAL REMEDIES TO KNOW

Cat's Claw:

Definition: Cat's claw, scientifically known as Uncaria tomentosa, is a woody vine native to the Amazon rainforest and other parts of Central and South America. It has been used for centuries in traditional medicine by indigenous peoples for its potential health benefits.

Ingredients: Cat's claw contains various bioactive compounds, including alkaloids (such as oxindole alkaloids and quinovic acid glycosides), polyphenols, and other phytochemicals. These compounds are believed to contribute to the herb's medicinal properties, including its potential as an immune enhancer, anti-inflammatory, and antioxidant.

How to Prepare: Cat's claw is typically consumed as an herbal tea, tincture, or in supplement form (such as capsules or tablets). To make tea, dried cat's claw bark or leaves are steeped in hot water for several minutes before being strained and consumed.

Dosage: The appropriate dosage of cat's claw can vary depending on factors such as age, health status, and the specific preparation being used. It's important to follow the recommended dosage on the product label or consult with a qualified herbalist or healthcare professional for personalized guidance.

How to Use: Cat's claw tea, tincture, or supplements are typically taken orally. It's often used to support immune function, reduce inflammation, and promote overall well-being.

Side Effects: Cat's claw is generally considered safe for most people when used in moderate amounts. However, some individuals may experience mild side effects such as gastrointestinal upset or allergic reactions. It may also interact with certain medications or have adverse effects in individuals with certain health conditions, such as autoimmune diseases or bleeding disorders. Pregnant or breastfeeding individuals should consult with a healthcare professional before using cat's claw supplements. It's important to use cat's claw under the guidance of a healthcare professional and to discontinue use if any adverse effects occur.

Chickweed:

Definition: Chickweed, scientifically known as Stellaria media, is an annual herbaceous plant native to Europe but naturalized in many other parts of the world. It's often considered a common weed but has been used historically in traditional medicine for its potential health benefits.

Ingredients: Chickweed contains various bioactive compounds, including flavonoids, saponins, mucilage, and vitamins (such as vitamin C). These compounds are believed to contribute to the herb's medicinal properties, including its potential as a demulcent, anti-inflammatory, and mild diuretic.

How to Prepare: Chickweed is typically consumed as an herbal tea, infusion, or in fresh salads. To make tea, dried chickweed leaves and flowers are steeped in hot water for several minutes before being strained and consumed. It can also be used topically as a poultice or infused oil for skin conditions.

Dosage: The appropriate dosage of chickweed can vary depending on factors such as age, health status, and the specific preparation being used. It's important to follow the recommended dosage on the product label or consult with a qualified herbalist or healthcare professional for personalized guidance.

How to Use: Chickweed tea, infusion, or fresh leaves are typically taken orally. It's often used to soothe inflammation, support digestion, and promote overall well-being. Topically, chickweed can be applied to the skin to alleviate itching, irritation, or minor wounds.

Side Effects: Chickweed is generally considered safe for most people when consumed in moderate amounts. However, some individuals may experience allergic reactions or gastrointestinal upset. It may also interact with certain medications or have adverse effects in individuals with certain health conditions. Pregnant or breastfeeding individuals should consult with a healthcare professional before using chickweed supplements. It's important to use chickweed under the guidance of a healthcare professional and to discontinue use if any adverse effects occur.

Cleavers:

Definition: Cleavers, scientifically known as Galium aparine, is a herbaceous annual plant native to Europe, North America, Asia, and Australia. It has a long history of use in traditional medicine for its potential health benefits.

Ingredients: Cleavers contains various bioactive compounds, including iridoid glycosides, flavonoids, tannins, and mucilage. These compounds are believed to contribute to the herb's medicinal properties, including its potential as a diuretic, lymphatic tonic, and mild astringent.

How to Prepare: Cleavers is typically consumed as an herbal tea, infusion, or in fresh salads. To make tea, dried cleavers leaves and stems are steeped in hot water for several minutes before being strained and consumed. It can also be used topically as a poultice or infused oil for skin conditions.

Dosage: The appropriate dosage of cleavers can vary depending on factors such as age, health status, and the specific preparation being used. It's important to follow the recommended dosage on the product label or consult with a qualified herbalist or healthcare professional for personalized guidance.

How to Use: Cleavers tea, infusion, or fresh leaves are typically taken orally. It's often used to support lymphatic drainage, promote urinary tract health, and soothe inflammation. Topically, cleavers can be applied to the skin to alleviate itching, irritation, or minor wounds.

Side Effects: Cleavers is generally considered safe for most people when consumed in moderate amounts. However, some individuals may experience allergic reactions or gastrointestinal upset. It may also interact with certain medications or have adverse effects in individuals with certain health conditions. Pregnant or breastfeeding individuals should consult with a healthcare professional before using cleavers supplements. It's important to use cleavers under the guidance of a healthcare professional and to discontinue use if any adverse effects occur.

Eucalyptus:

Definition: Eucalyptus refers to a genus of flowering trees and shrubs, primarily native to Australia but also found in other parts of the world. Eucalyptus essential oil, extracted from the leaves of certain species, has a long history of use in traditional medicine for its potential health benefits.

Ingredients: Eucalyptus essential oil contains various bioactive compounds, including eucalyptol (cineole), terpenes, and flavonoids. These compounds are believed to contribute to the oil's medicinal properties, including its potential as an expectorant, decongestant, antiseptic, and anti-inflammatory.

How to Prepare: Eucalyptus essential oil can be used in aromatherapy, diffused in the air, or diluted and applied topically to the skin. It can also be added to steam inhalations or chest rubs to help relieve respiratory symptoms.

Dosage: The appropriate dosage of eucalyptus essential oil can vary depending on factors such as age, health status, and the specific application being used. It's important to follow the recommended dosage on the product label or consult with a qualified aromatherapist or healthcare professional for personalized guidance.

How to Use: Eucalyptus essential oil can be used aromatically, topically, or internally, depending on the intended application. It's often used to alleviate respiratory congestion, soothe sore muscles, promote relaxation, and support overall well-being.

Side Effects: Eucalyptus essential oil is generally considered safe for most people when used appropriately. However, it can be toxic if ingested in large amounts and should not be applied directly to the skin without proper dilution. Some individuals may experience allergic reactions or respiratory irritation when exposed to eucalyptus oil. It's important to use eucalyptus oil with caution, especially around children and pets. Pregnant or breastfeeding individuals should consult with a healthcare professional before using eucalyptus oil. If any adverse effects occur, discontinue use and seek medical attention.

Feverfew:

Definition: Feverfew, scientifically known as Tanacetum parthenium, is a perennial herb native to Europe but also found in other parts of the world. It has a long history of use in traditional medicine, particularly in European folk medicine, for its potential health benefits.

Ingredients: Feverfew contains various bioactive compounds, including sesquiterpene lactones (such as parthenolide), flavonoids, and volatile oils. These compounds are believed to contribute to the herb's medicinal properties, including its potential as an anti-inflammatory, analgesic, and migraine prophylactic.

How to Prepare: Feverfew is typically consumed as an herbal tea, tincture, or in supplement form (such as capsules or tablets). To make tea, dried feverfew leaves and flowers are steeped in hot water for several minutes before being strained and consumed.

Dosage: The appropriate dosage of feverfew can vary depending on factors such as age, health status, and the specific preparation being used. It's important to follow the recommended dosage on the product label or consult with a qualified herbalist or healthcare professional for personalized guidance.

How to Use: Feverfew tea, tincture, or supplements are typically taken orally. It's often used to alleviate headaches, including migraines, and to support overall well-being.

Side Effects: Feverfew is generally considered safe for most people when used in moderate amounts. However, some individuals may experience mild side effects such as gastrointestinal upset or allergic reactions. It may also interact with certain medications or have adverse effects in individuals with certain health conditions, such as bleeding disorders or pregnancy. It's important to use feverfew under the guidance of a healthcare professional and to discontinue use if any adverse effects occur.

Ginseng:

Definition: Ginseng refers to several species of perennial plants belonging to the Panax genus, including Panax ginseng (Asian ginseng) and Panax quinquefolius (American ginseng). Ginseng has been used for centuries in traditional medicine, particularly in East Asia, for its potential health benefits.

Ingredients: Ginseng root contains various bioactive compounds, including ginsenosides, polysaccharides, and peptides. These compounds are believed to contribute to the herb's medicinal properties, including its potential as an adaptogen, immune enhancer, and cognitive booster.

How to Prepare: Ginseng is typically consumed as a powdered root, herbal tea, tincture, or in supplement form (such as capsules or tablets). To make tea, dried ginseng root slices are simmered in water for several minutes before being strained and consumed.

Dosage: The appropriate dosage of ginseng can vary depending on factors such as age, health status, and the specific preparation being used. It's important to follow the recommended dosage on the product label or consult with a qualified herbalist or healthcare professional for personalized guidance.

How to Use: Ginseng powder, tea, tincture, or supplements are typically taken orally. It's often used to support energy levels, enhance cognitive function, and promote overall well-being.

Side Effects: Ginseng is generally considered safe for most people when used in moderate amounts. However, some individuals may experience mild side effects such as insomnia, gastrointestinal upset, or headaches. It may also interact with certain medications or have adverse effects in individuals with certain health conditions, such as high blood pressure or diabetes. Pregnant or breastfeeding individuals should consult with a healthcare professional before using ginseng supplements. It's important to use ginseng under the guidance of a healthcare professional and to discontinue use if any adverse effects occur.

Goldenseal:

Definition: Goldenseal, scientifically known as Hydrastis canadensis, is a perennial herb native to North America. It has a long history of use in traditional Native American medicine and later in folk medicine for its potential health benefits.

Ingredients: Goldenseal root contains various bioactive compounds, including alkaloids (such as berberine and hydrastine), flavonoids, and volatile oils. These compounds are believed to contribute to the herb's medicinal properties, including its potential as an antimicrobial, anti-inflammatory, and immune enhancer.

How to Prepare: Goldenseal is typically consumed as an herbal tea, tincture, or in supplement form (such as capsules or tablets). To make tea, dried goldenseal root or leaves are steeped in hot water for several minutes before being strained and consumed.

Dosage: The appropriate dosage of goldenseal can vary depending on factors such as age, health status, and the specific preparation being used. It's important to follow the recommended dosage on the product label or consult with a qualified herbalist or healthcare professional for personalized guidance.

How to Use: Goldenseal tea, tincture, or supplements are typically taken orally. It's often used to support immune function, promote digestive health, and soothe inflammation.

Side Effects: Goldenseal is generally considered safe for most people when used in moderate amounts. However, some individuals may experience mild side effects such as gastrointestinal upset or allergic reactions. It may also interact with certain medications or have adverse effects in individuals with certain health conditions, such as high blood pressure or pregnancy. It's important to use goldenseal under the guidance of a healthcare professional and to discontinue use if any adverse effects occur.

Bio Ferro Tonic:

Definition: Bio Ferro Tonic is a dietary supplement primarily composed of herbs and minerals. It's often marketed as a natural way to support overall health, particularly by promoting blood health and circulation.

Ingredients: Typical ingredients in Bio Ferro Tonic may include a blend of herbs such as burdock root, yellow dock root, sarsaparilla root, and cascara sagrada bark, along with minerals like iron and potassium phosphate.

How to Prepare: Bio Ferro Tonic usually comes in liquid form and is typically taken orally. It's important to follow the instructions on the product label for dosage and administration.

Dosage: The dosage can vary depending on the specific product and individual needs. It's crucial to consult with a healthcare professional or follow the recommended dosage on the product label to avoid potential side effects.

How to Use: Bio Ferro Tonic is often taken by adding the recommended dosage to water or juice and consuming it orally. It's important to shake the bottle well before use and store it according to the manufacturer's instructions.

Side Effects: While Bio Ferro Tonic is generally considered safe when used as directed, some individuals may experience side effects such as digestive discomfort, allergic reactions, or interactions with medications. It's essential to consult with a healthcare provider before starting any new supplement regimen, especially if you have underlying health conditions or are taking medications.

Bladderwrack:

Definition: Bladderwrack is a type of seaweed or marine algae commonly used in traditional medicine and as a dietary supplement. It's known for its potential health benefits, particularly related to thyroid health and weight management.

Ingredients: Bladderwrack contains various nutrients, including iodine, vitamins, minerals, and antioxidants. The primary active components are iodine and fucoidan, a type of carbohydrate found in brown seaweeds.

How to Prepare: Bladderwrack supplements are available in various forms, including capsules, powders, and liquid extracts. They can be taken orally with water or added to smoothies and other beverages.

Dosage: The appropriate dosage of bladderwrack can vary based on factors such as age, health status, and the specific product being used. It's essential to follow the recommended dosage on the product label or consult with a healthcare professional for personalized guidance.

How to Use: Bladderwrack supplements are typically taken orally, either with water or mixed into food or beverages. It's important to follow the instructions on the product label and avoid exceeding the recommended dosage.

Side Effects: While bladderwrack is generally considered safe for most people when used in moderation, excessive intake of iodine from bladderwrack supplements can cause thyroid dysfunction and other adverse effects. Individuals with thyroid disorders, iodine sensitivity, or certain medical conditions should exercise caution and consult with a healthcare provider before using bladderwrack supplements. Common side effects may include digestive upset, allergic reactions, or interactions with medications.

Blood Purifier:

Definition: Blood purifiers are herbal remedies or dietary supplements believed to cleanse or detoxify the blood, often promoting overall health and well-being. They are thought to support the body's natural detoxification processes and improve blood circulation.

Ingredients: Blood purifiers may contain a variety of herbs and botanical extracts known for their purported cleansing and detoxifying properties. Common ingredients include burdock root, red clover, dandelion root, and yellow dock root, among others.

How to Prepare: Blood purifiers are typically available in various forms, including capsules, tablets, powders, and liquid extracts. They are usually taken orally with water or juice, following the recommended dosage on the product label.

Dosage: The dosage of blood purifiers can vary depending on the specific product and individual needs. It's important to adhere to the recommended dosage on the product label or consult with a healthcare professional for personalized guidance.

How to Use: Blood purifiers are typically taken orally, either with water or mixed into beverages. They are often used as part of a detoxification regimen or to support overall health and vitality.

Side Effects: While blood purifiers are generally considered safe for most people when used as directed, some individuals may experience side effects such as digestive discomfort, allergic reactions, or interactions with medications. It's important to consult with a healthcare provider before starting any new supplement regimen, especially if you have underlying health conditions or are taking medications.

Blue Vervain:

Definition: Blue vervain, also known as Verbena hastata, is a perennial herb native to North America. It has been used in traditional medicine for centuries to treat various ailments, including anxiety, insomnia, and digestive issues.

Ingredients: Blue vervain contains several active compounds, including aucubin, verbenalin, and volatile oils. These compounds are believed to contribute to the herb's medicinal properties.

How to Prepare: Blue vervain is typically consumed as a tea or tincture. To make tea, dried blue vervain leaves and flowers are steeped in hot water for several minutes before being strained and consumed. Tinctures are prepared by steeping the herb in alcohol or vinegar to extract its active compounds.

Dosage: The appropriate dosage of blue vervain can vary depending on factors such as age, health status, and the specific preparation being used. It's important to follow the recommended dosage on the product label or consult with a qualified herbalist or healthcare professional for personalized guidance.

How to Use: Blue vervain tea or tincture is typically taken orally. It can be consumed on its own or mixed with honey or other herbal teas for added flavor.

Side Effects: While blue vervain is generally considered safe for most people when used in moderation, excessive intake may cause digestive upset or allergic reactions in some individuals. Pregnant or breastfeeding women should avoid blue vervain due to its potential to stimulate uterine contractions. As with any herbal remedy, it's important to consult with a healthcare provider before using blue vervain, especially if you have underlying health conditions or are taking medications.

Bromide Plus Powder:

Definition: Bromide Plus Powder is a dietary supplement formulated to support thyroid health and promote overall well-being. It typically contains a blend of herbs and minerals that are believed to have beneficial effects on thyroid function.

Ingredients: Bromide Plus Powder often contains a combination of herbs such as bladderwrack, sea moss, and burdock root, along with minerals like iodine and potassium phosphate. These ingredients are thought to support thyroid function and maintain optimal iodine levels in the body.

How to Prepare: Bromide Plus Powder is usually mixed with water or juice to create a drinkable solution. It's important to follow the instructions on the product label for dosage and preparation.

Dosage: The dosage of Bromide Plus Powder can vary depending on the specific product and individual needs. It's crucial to consult with a healthcare professional or follow the recommended dosage on the product label to avoid potential side effects.

How to Use: Bromide Plus Powder is typically taken orally by mixing the recommended dosage with water or juice. It's important to shake or stir the mixture well before consuming it to ensure even distribution of the ingredients.

Side Effects: While Bromide Plus Powder is generally considered safe when used as directed, some individuals may experience side effects such as digestive discomfort or allergic reactions to certain ingredients. It's essential to consult with a healthcare provider before starting any new supplement regimen, especially if you have underlying health conditions or are taking medications.

Bugleweed:

Definition: Bugleweed, also known as Lycopusvirginicus, is a perennial herb native to North America and Europe. It has been used in traditional medicine to treat various conditions, including hyperthyroidism, anxiety, and insomnia.

Ingredients: Bugleweed contains several active compounds, including lithospermic acid, phenolic acids, and flavonoids. These compounds are believed to contribute to the herb's medicinal properties, particularly its ability to regulate thyroid function.

How to Prepare: Bugleweed is commonly consumed as a tea or tincture. To make tea, dried bugleweed leaves and flowers are steeped in hot water for several minutes before being strained and consumed. Tinctures are prepared by steeping the herb in alcohol or vinegar to extract its active compounds.

Dosage: The appropriate dosage of bugleweed can vary depending on factors such as age, health status, and the specific preparation being used. It's important to follow the recommended dosage on the product label or consult with a qualified herbalist or healthcare professional for personalized guidance.

How to Use: Bugleweed tea or tincture is typically taken orally. It can be consumed on its own or mixed with honey or other herbal teas for added flavor.

Side Effects: While bugleweed is generally considered safe for most people when used in moderation, excessive intake may cause digestive upset or allergic reactions in some individuals. Pregnant or breastfeeding women should avoid bugleweed due to its potential to stimulate uterine contractions. As with any herbal remedy, it's important to consult with a healthcare provider before using bugleweed, especially if you have underlying health conditions or are taking medications.

Burdock:

Definition: Burdock, scientifically known as Arctium lappa, is a biennial plant native to Europe and Asia but now found worldwide. It's part of the Asteraceae family and has been used for centuries in traditional medicine and culinary practices.

Ingredients: Burdock contains various nutrients, including carbohydrates, fiber, vitamins (such as vitamin B6, folate, and vitamin C), and minerals (including potassium, magnesium, and manganese). It also contains active compounds such as polyphenols and volatile oils.

How to Prepare: Burdock can be prepared and consumed in various ways. The roots, leaves, and seeds are all utilized for different purposes. The root is commonly used in cooking, herbal teas, tinctures, and supplements, while the leaves and seeds are sometimes used in herbal preparations.

Dosage: The appropriate dosage of burdock root can vary depending on the specific form and intended use. For culinary purposes, there are no strict dosage guidelines, but for supplements or herbal remedies, it's essential to follow the recommended dosage on the product label or consult with a healthcare professional.

How to Use: Burdock root can be used in cooking by peeling, slicing, and adding it to soups, stews, stir-fries, or salads. It can also be brewed into a tea or used to make tinctures or extracts for medicinal purposes. Some people may also take burdock root supplements in capsule or powder form.

Side Effects: While burdock is generally considered safe for most people when consumed in moderate amounts, some individuals may experience allergic reactions or digestive upset. Additionally, burdock may interact with certain medications or have adverse effects in individuals with certain health conditions, such as diabetes or allergies to plants in the Asteraceae family. It's important to consult with a healthcare provider before using burdock, especially if you have underlying health conditions or are taking medications.

Cascara Sagrada:

Definition: Cascara Sagrada, scientifically known as Rhamnus purshiana, is a species of buckthorn native to western North America. It has been used traditionally as a laxative and to promote bowel regularity.

Ingredients: The primary active ingredients in cascara sagrada are anthraquinone glycosides, particularly cascarosides A and B. These compounds stimulate peristalsis in the colon, leading to increased bowel movements.

How to Prepare: Cascara sagrada is typically prepared as an herbal tea, tincture, or capsule. To make tea, dried cascara sagrada bark is steeped in hot water for several minutes before being strained and consumed. Tinctures are prepared by steeping the bark in alcohol to extract its active compounds.

Dosage: The appropriate dosage of cascara sagrada can vary depending on the specific preparation and intended use. It's important to follow the recommended dosage on the product label or consult with a healthcare professional for personalized guidance.

How to Use: Cascara sagrada tea or tincture is typically taken orally. It's important to start with a low dose and gradually increase if needed to avoid potential side effects such as cramping or diarrhea.

Side Effects: Cascara sagrada is considered safe for short-term use when used as directed. However, long-term or excessive use may lead to dependence, electrolyte imbalance, or dehydration. It may also interact with certain medications or have adverse effects in individuals with certain health conditions. It's important to use cascara sagrada under the guidance of a healthcare professional and to discontinue use if any adverse effects occur.

Cell Food:

Definition: Cell Food is a dietary supplement marketed as a highly oxygenating and alkalizing formula. It's claimed to support overall health and vitality by providing essential nutrients and oxygen to the cells.

Ingredients: The exact ingredients of Cell Food can vary depending on the brand, but it typically contains a proprietary blend of minerals, enzymes, electrolytes, and trace elements. Some common ingredients may include purified water, dissolved oxygen, seawater extract, and plant-based enzymes.

How to Prepare: Cell Food is usually available in liquid form and is typically taken orally. It can be consumed directly or diluted in water or juice before consumption.

Dosage: The dosage of Cell Food can vary depending on the specific product and individual needs. It's important to follow the recommended dosage on the product label or consult with a healthcare professional for personalized guidance.

How to Use: Cell Food is typically taken orally, either directly or mixed into water or juice. It's important to shake the bottle well before use and to store it according to the manufacturer's instructions.

Side Effects: Cell Food is generally considered safe for most people when used as directed. However, some individuals may experience mild digestive upset or allergic reactions to certain ingredients. It's essential to consult with a healthcare provider before starting any new supplement regimen, especially if you have underlying health conditions or are taking medications.

Chaparral:

Definition: Chaparral, scientifically known as Larrea tridentata, is a shrub native to the southwestern United States and northern Mexico. It has been used for centuries by Native American tribes for its medicinal properties and is commonly used in herbal medicine today.

Ingredients: Chaparral contains several bioactive compounds, including nordihydroguaiaretic acid (NDGA), flavonoids, lignans, and volatile oils. NDGA is believed to be the primary active compound responsible for many of chaparral's therapeutic effects.

How to Prepare: Chaparral can be prepared and consumed in various forms, including teas, tinctures, capsules, and topical preparations. To make tea, dried chaparral leaves are steeped in hot water for several minutes before being strained and consumed. Tinctures are prepared by steeping the herb in alcohol or vinegar to extract its active compounds.

Dosage: The appropriate dosage of chaparral can vary depending on the specific form and intended use. It's important to follow the recommended dosage on the product label or consult with a healthcare professional for personalized guidance.

How to Use: Chaparral tea or tincture is typically taken orally. It can also be applied topically to the skin for certain conditions. It's important to use chaparral products as directed and to discontinue use if any adverse effects occur.

Side Effects: Chaparral is generally considered safe for most people when used in moderate amounts. However, excessive intake or prolonged use may lead to liver toxicity or other adverse effects. It may also interact with certain medications or have adverse effects in individuals with certain health conditions. It's important to use chaparral under the guidance of a healthcare professional and to discontinue use if any adverse effects occur.

Cocolmeca:

Definition: Cocolmeca, also known as Smilax ornata or sarsaparilla, is a flowering vine native to Mexico and Central America. It has been used traditionally in Mexican and Central American folk medicine for its purported medicinal properties.

Ingredients: Cocolmeca contains various bioactive compounds, including saponins, flavonoids, and plant sterols. These compounds are believed to contribute to the herb's medicinal properties, including its potential as a diuretic, blood purifier, and anti-inflammatory agent.

How to Prepare: Cocolmeca is commonly prepared and consumed as an herbal tea or decoction. To make tea, dried cocolmeca roots or leaves are steeped in hot water for several minutes before being strained and consumed. Decoctions involve boiling the roots or leaves in water to extract their active compounds.

Dosage: The appropriate dosage of cocolmeca can vary depending on factors such as age, health status, and the specific preparation being used. It's important to follow the recommended dosage on the product label or consult with a qualified herbalist or healthcare professional for personalized guidance.

How to Use: Cocolmeca tea or decoction is typically taken orally. It can also be used topically for certain skin conditions. It's important to use cocolmeca products as directed and to discontinue use if any adverse effects occur.

Side Effects: Cocolmeca is generally considered safe for most people when used in moderate amounts. However, excessive intake may lead to digestive upset or other adverse effects. It may also interact with certain medications or have adverse effects in individuals with certain health conditions. It's important to use cocolmeca under the guidance of a healthcare professional and to discontinue use if any adverse effects occur.

Contribo:

Definition: Contribo, also known as Aristolochiatrilobata, is a vine native to the Caribbean and Central America. It has been used traditionally in folk medicine for various purposes, including as a remedy for digestive issues, inflammation, and pain relief.

Ingredients: Contribo contains several bioactive compounds, including aristolochic acids, flavonoids, and alkaloids. These compounds are believed to contribute to the herb's medicinal properties, including its potential as an anti-inflammatory and analgesic agent.

How to Prepare: Contribo is typically prepared and consumed as an herbal tea or decoction. To make tea, dried contribo leaves or stems are steeped in hot water for several minutes before being strained and consumed. Decoctions involve boiling the leaves or stems in water to extract their active compounds.

Dosage: The appropriate dosage of contribo can vary depending on factors such as age, health status, and the specific preparation being used. It's important to follow the recommended dosage on the product label or consult with a qualified herbalist or healthcare professional for personalized guidance.

How to Use: Contribo tea or decoction is typically taken orally. It's important to use contribo products as directed and to discontinue use if any adverse effects occur.

Side Effects: Contribo contains aristolochic acids, which have been associated with serious adverse effects, including kidney damage and cancer. Due to these safety concerns, the use of contribo is highly discouraged, and it's important to avoid products containing aristolochic acids. Individuals should seek alternative remedies for their health needs.

Dandelion Root:

Definition: Dandelion, scientifically known as Taraxacum officinale, is a common flowering plant found worldwide. While often considered a pesky weed, dandelion has a long history of use in traditional medicine for its various health benefits.

Ingredients: Dandelion root contains several bioactive compounds, including sesquiterpene lactones, triterpenes, flavonoids, and polysaccharides. These compounds are believed to contribute to the herb's medicinal properties, including its potential as a diuretic, digestive aid, and liver tonic.

How to Prepare: Dandelion root can be prepared and consumed in various forms, including teas, tinctures, capsules, and extracts. To make tea, dried dandelion root is steeped in hot water for several minutes before being strained and consumed. Tinctures are prepared by steeping the root in alcohol or vinegar to extract its active compounds.

Dosage: The appropriate dosage of dandelion root can vary depending on factors such as age, health status, and the specific preparation being used. It's important to follow the recommended dosage on the product label or consult with a qualified herbalist or healthcare professional for personalized guidance.

How to Use: Dandelion root tea, tincture, or capsules are typically taken orally. It's important to use dandelion root products as directed and to discontinue use if any adverse effects occur.

Side Effects: Dandelion root is generally considered safe for most people when used in moderate amounts. However, some individuals may experience allergic reactions or digestive upset. It may also interact with certain medications or have adverse effects in individuals with certain health conditions. It's important to use dandelion root under the guidance of a healthcare professional and to discontinue use if any adverse effects occur.

Green Food Plus:

Definition: Green Food Plus is a dietary supplement formulated to provide a concentrated source of nutrients derived from various green plants. It's designed to support overall health and well-being by delivering essential vitamins, minerals, antioxidants, and phytonutrients.

Ingredients: Green Food Plus typically contains a blend of powdered green vegetables, grasses, algae, and other plant-based ingredients. Common ingredients may include wheatgrass, barley grass, spirulina, chlorella, alfalfa, kale, spinach, and broccoli, among others.

How to Prepare: Green Food Plus is usually available in powder form and can be mixed with water, juice, or smoothies. It's important to follow the recommended dosage on the product label and to consume it as part of a balanced diet.

Dosage: The appropriate dosage of Green Food Plus can vary depending on the specific product and individual needs. It's important to follow the recommended dosage on the product label or consult with a healthcare professional for personalized guidance.

How to Use: Green Food Plus powder is typically mixed with water, juice, or smoothies and consumed orally. It's often taken once or twice daily, preferably with meals, to maximize nutrient absorption.

Side Effects: Green Food Plus is generally considered safe for most people when used as directed. However, some individuals may experience digestive upset or allergic reactions to certain ingredients. It's important to consult with a healthcare provider before starting any new supplement regimen, especially if you have underlying health conditions or are taking medications.

Hops:

Definition: Hops, scientifically known as Humulus lupulus, is a perennial climbing vine native to Europe, Asia, and North America. It is primarily known for its use in brewing beer but has also been used historically in traditional medicine for its potential health benefits.

Ingredients: Hops flowers contain various bioactive compounds, including bitter acids (such as humulone and lupulone), essential oils, flavonoids, and polyphenols. These compounds are believed to contribute to the herb's medicinal properties, including its potential as a sedative, relaxant, and digestive aid.

How to Prepare: Hops is typically consumed as an herbal tea, tincture, or in supplement form (such as capsules or tablets). To make tea, dried hops flowers are steeped in hot water for several minutes before being strained and consumed.

Dosage: The appropriate dosage of hops can vary depending on factors such as age, health status, and the specific preparation being used. It's important to follow the recommended dosage on the product label or consult with a qualified herbalist or healthcare professional for personalized guidance.

How to Use: Hops tea, tincture, or supplements are typically taken orally. It's often used to promote relaxation, relieve anxiety, and support sleep.

Side Effects: Hops is generally considered safe for most people when used in moderate amounts. However, some individuals may experience mild side effects such as drowsiness, gastrointestinal upset, or allergic reactions. It may also interact with certain medications or have adverse effects in individuals with certain health conditions, such as depression or hormone-sensitive conditions. It's important to use hops under the guidance of a healthcare professional and to discontinue use if any adverse effects occur.

Kelp:

Definition: Kelp refers to several species of large brown algae belonging to the Laminariales order. It is commonly found in underwater forests along rocky coastlines around the world. Kelp has been used for centuries in various cultures, particularly in East Asia, for its nutritional and medicinal properties.

Ingredients: Kelp is rich in various nutrients, including iodine, vitamins (such as vitamin K, vitamin C, and B vitamins), minerals (including calcium, magnesium, and potassium), antioxidants, and fiber. These nutrients are believed to contribute to the seaweed's potential health benefits, including its role in thyroid function, bone health, and immune support.

How to Prepare: Kelp is typically consumed dried, powdered, or in supplement form (such as capsules or tablets). It can also be used in cooking, particularly in soups, salads, and stir-fries. Kelp supplements are available in various forms, including powdered extracts, tablets, and liquid extracts.

Dosage: The appropriate dosage of kelp can vary depending on factors such as age, health status, and the specific preparation being used. It's important to follow the recommended dosage on the product label or consult with a qualified healthcare professional for personalized guidance.

How to Use: Kelp supplements are typically taken orally with water. They can be consumed as part of a daily nutritional regimen to support overall health and well-being. Kelp can also be incorporated into recipes as a flavorful and nutritious ingredient.

Side Effects: While kelp is generally considered safe for most people when consumed in moderate amounts, excessive intake of iodine-rich foods or supplements, including kelp, can lead to thyroid dysfunction or iodine toxicity. Some individuals may also be allergic to seaweed and experience allergic reactions. Pregnant or breastfeeding individuals should consult with a healthcare professional before using kelp supplements. It's important to use kelp under the guidance of a healthcare professional and to discontinue use if any adverse effects occur.

Astragalus:

Definition: Astragalus, scientifically known as Astragalus membranaceus, is a flowering plant native to China and Mongolia but also found in other parts of Asia. It has been used for centuries in traditional Chinese medicine for its potential health benefits, particularly for its immune-enhancing properties.

Ingredients: Astragalus root contains various bioactive compounds, including polysaccharides, saponins (such as astragalosides), flavonoids, and amino acids. These compounds are believed to contribute to the herb's medicinal properties, including its potential as an adaptogen, immunomodulator, and anti-inflammatory agent.

How to Prepare: Astragalus is typically consumed as a powdered root, herbal tea, tincture, or in supplement form (such as capsules or tablets). To make tea, dried astragalus root slices are simmered in water for several minutes before being strained and consumed.

Dosage: The appropriate dosage of astragalus can vary depending on factors such as age, health status, and the specific preparation being used. It's important to follow the recommended dosage on the product label or consult with a qualified herbalist or healthcare professional for personalized guidance.

How to Use: Astragalus powder, tea, tincture, or supplements are typically taken orally. It's often consumed to support immune function, promote vitality, and enhance overall well-being.

Side Effects: Astragalus is generally considered safe for most people when used in moderate amounts. However, some individuals may experience mild side effects such as gastrointestinal upset or allergic reactions. It may also interact with certain medications or have adverse effects in individuals with certain health conditions, such as autoimmune diseases or diabetes. Pregnant or breastfeeding individuals should consult with a healthcare professional before using astragalus supplements. It's important to use astragalus under the guidance of a healthcare professional and to discontinue use if any adverse effects occur.

Black Cohosh:

Definition: Black cohosh, scientifically known as Actaea racemosa (formerly Cimicifuga racemosa), is a perennial herb native to North America. It has a long history of use in traditional Native American medicine and later in folk medicine for its potential health benefits, particularly for women's health.

Ingredients: Black cohosh root contains various bioactive compounds, including triterpene glycosides (such as actein and cimicifugoside), phenolic acids, and flavonoids. These compounds are believed to contribute to the herb's medicinal properties, including its potential as a hormone-balancing agent and its ability to relieve menopausal symptoms.

How to Prepare: Black cohosh is typically consumed as a powdered root, herbal tea, tincture, or in supplement form (such as capsules or tablets). To make tea, dried black cohosh root is steeped in hot water for several minutes before being strained and consumed.

Dosage: The appropriate dosage of black cohosh can vary depending on factors such as age, health status, and the specific preparation being used. It's important to follow the recommended dosage on the product label or consult with a qualified herbalist or healthcare professional for personalized guidance.

How to Use: Black cohosh powder, tea, tincture, or supplements are typically taken orally. It's often used by women to support hormonal balance, relieve menopausal symptoms such as hot flashes and night sweats, and promote overall well-being.

Side Effects: Black cohosh is generally considered safe for most people when used in moderate amounts. However, some individuals may experience mild side effects such as gastrointestinal upset or allergic reactions. It may also interact with certain medications or have adverse effects in individuals with certain health conditions, such as liver disease or hormone-sensitive conditions. Pregnant or breastfeeding individuals should consult with a healthcare professional before using black cohosh supplements. It's important to use black cohosh under the guidance of a healthcare professional and to discontinue use if any adverse effects occur.

Blessed Thistle:

Definition: Blessed thistle, scientifically known as Cnicusbenedictus, is an annual or biennial herb native to the Mediterranean region but also found in other parts of Europe, Asia, and North Africa. It has been used historically in traditional medicine for its potential health benefits, particularly for digestive and liver health.

Ingredients: Blessed thistle contains various bioactive compounds, including sesquiterpene lactones (such as cnicin), flavonoids, tannins, and essential oils. These compounds are believed to contribute to the herb's medicinal properties, including its potential as a digestive tonic, appetite stimulant, and liver tonic.

How to Prepare: Blessed thistle is typically consumed as an herbal tea, tincture, or in supplement form (such as capsules or tablets). To make tea, dried blessed thistle leaves and flowers are steeped in hot water for several minutes before being strained and consumed.

Dosage: The appropriate dosage of blessed thistle can vary depending on factors such as age, health status, and the specific preparation being used. It's important to follow the recommended dosage on the product label or consult with a qualified herbalist or healthcare professional for personalized guidance.

How to Use: Blessed thistle tea, tincture, or supplements are typically taken orally. It's often used to support digestion, stimulate appetite, and promote liver health.

Side Effects: Blessed thistle is generally considered safe for most people when used in moderate amounts. However, some individuals may experience mild side effects such as gastrointestinal upset or allergic reactions. It may also interact with certain medications or have adverse effects in individuals with certain health conditions, such as hormone-sensitive conditions or bleeding disorders. Pregnant or breastfeeding individuals should consult with a healthcare professional before using blessed thistle supplements. It's important to use blessed thistle under the guidance of a healthcare professional and to discontinue use if any adverse effects occur.

THE END